The Complete Noom Diet Cookbook

100+ Delicious Recipes for Healthy Living and Weight Loss with the NOOM Diet

By Dr. Melissa Clark

Table of Contents

Introduction

Welcome to "The Complete NOOM DIET Cookbook"! This cookbook is designed to be your ultimate companion on your journey towards a healthier and happier you. Whether you're new to the NOOM Diet or a seasoned enthusiast, you'll find a wealth of delicious and nutritious recipes that align perfectly with the principles of this popular and effective weight management program.

The NOOM Diet is not just another diet; it's a lifestyle change that focuses on sustainable, mindful eating. It emphasizes the importance of making informed food choices, being aware of portion sizes, and cultivating a positive relationship with food. Instead of strict rules and restrictions, the NOOM Diet encourages you to make healthier choices and build better habits over time.

To make your cooking journey as easy and enjoyable as possible, we've included detailed instructions, ingredient lists, and nutritional information for each recipe. We believe that cooking should be a joyful experience, and we hope these recipes inspire you to get creative in the kitchen while staying on track with your health goals.

Remember, the NOOM Diet is all about balance and making sustainable choices that work for you. It's not about depriving yourself or feeling guilty about the foods you enjoy. Instead, it's about making mindful choices, understanding your eating habits, and achieving a healthier relationship with food.

So, grab your apron, get ready to explore these delicious recipes, and embark on a journey toward a healthier and happier you with "The Complete NOOM DIET Cookbook" as your trusted guide. Here's to a future filled with flavorful, nutritious meals that support your well-being!

Chapter 1: Breakfast Delights

Greek Yogurt Parfait

Cook time: 5 minutes

Serving: 1

Ingredients:

- 1/2 cup plain Greek yogurt
- 1/4 cup fresh berries (such as strawberries, blueberries, or blackberries)
- 1/4 cup granola
- 1 tablespoon honey

Preparation:

1. In a small bowl, layer the Greek yogurt, fresh berries, and granola.
2. Drizzle honey on top of the parfait.
3. Enjoy immediately or store in the fridge for later.

Oatmeal with Fresh Berries

Cook time: 10 minutes

Serving: 1

Ingredients:

- 1/2 cup rolled oats
- 1 cup water or milk
- 1/4 cup fresh berries
- 1 tablespoon honey or maple syrup
- 1 tablespoon chopped nuts (optional)

Preparation:

1. In a small pot, bring the water or milk to a boil.
2. Add in the rolled oats and reduce to a simmer for 5-7 minutes, stirring occasionally.
3. Once the oats are cooked, remove from heat and let sit for 2-3 minutes.
4. Add in the fresh berries, honey or maple syrup, and chopped nuts (if using).
5. Stir to combine and enjoy.

Veggie Omelette

Cook time: 15 minutes

Serving: 1

Ingredients:

- 2 large eggs
- 1/4 cup chopped vegetables (such as bell peppers, spinach, mushrooms, onions)
- 1 tablespoon shredded cheese
- Salt and pepper to taste
- 1 teaspoon butter or oil

Preparation:

1. In a small bowl, whisk together the eggs and salt and pepper.
2. In a nonstick pan, melt the butter or heat the oil over medium-high heat.
3. Add in the chopped vegetables and sauté for 2-3 minutes until slightly softened.
4. Pour the eggs over the vegetables and let cook for 2 minutes.
5. Use a spatula to lift the edges of the omelette and let the uncooked egg flow underneath.
6. Once the omelette is mostly cooked, sprinkle the shredded cheese on one half.
7. Use the spatula to carefully fold the other half of the omelette over the cheese.
8. Let cook for another minute until the cheese is melted and the eggs are fully cooked.
9. Slide the omelette onto a plate and serve hot.

Whole Grain Pancakes

Cook time: 20 minutes

Serving: 2

Ingredients:

- 1 cup whole grain flour
- 1 tablespoon baking powder
- 1 tablespoon honey or maple syrup
- 1/2 teaspoon salt
- 1 cup milk
- 1 large egg
- 1 tablespoon butter or oil

Preparation:

1. In a large bowl, whisk together the flour, baking powder, honey or maple syrup, and salt.
2. In a separate bowl, beat the egg and then stir in the milk.
3. Pour the wet ingredients into the dry ingredients and mix until just combined.
4. In a nonstick pan, melt the butter or heat the oil over medium-high heat.
5. Use a 1/4 cup measuring cup to pour the pancake batter onto the pan.
6. Cook for 2-3 minutes until bubbles form on the surface of the pancake and the edges look slightly dry.
7. Flip the pancake and cook for another 2 minutes until golden brown.
8. Repeat with the remaining batter.
9. Serve the pancakes with your choice of toppings, such as fresh fruit, honey or maple syrup, or nut butter.

Spinach and Mushroom Breakfast Quesadilla

Cook time: 15 minutes

Serving: 1

Ingredients:

- 2 small whole grain tortillas
- 1/4 cup shredded cheese
- 1/4 cup chopped spinach
- 1/4 cup sliced mushrooms
- 1 teaspoon butter or oil

Preparation:

1. In a nonstick pan, melt the butter or heat the oil over medium-high heat.
2. Place one tortilla in the pan and sprinkle half of the shredded cheese on top.
3. Add the chopped spinach and sliced mushrooms on top of the cheese.
4. Sprinkle the remaining cheese on top and cover with the second tortilla.
5. Cook for 2-3 minutes until the bottom tortilla is slightly crispy.
6. Carefully flip the quesadilla and cook for another 2-3 minutes until both sides are golden brown and the cheese is melted.
7. Slide the quesadilla onto a plate and cut into wedges.
8. Serve with salsa, hot sauce, or avocado on top.

Breakfast Burrito

Cook time: 10 minutes

Serving: 1

Ingredients:

- 1 large whole grain tortilla
- 2 large eggs
- 1/4 cup black beans, drained and rinsed
- 1/4 cup chopped bell peppers
- 2 tablespoons shredded cheese
- Salt and pepper to taste
- 1 teaspoon butter or oil

Preparation:

1. In a small bowl, whisk together the eggs and salt and pepper.
2. In a nonstick pan, melt the butter or heat the oil over medium-high heat.
3. Add in the chopped bell peppers and sauté for 2-3 minutes until slightly softened.
4. Pour the eggs over the bell peppers and let cook for 2 minutes.
5. Use a spatula to lift the edges of the eggs and let the uncooked egg flow underneath.
6. Once the eggs are mostly cooked, add in the drained black beans and shredded cheese on one half of the eggs.
7. Fold the other half of the eggs over the beans and cheese.
8. Use the spatula to carefully transfer the burrito onto a tortilla.
9. Roll up the tortilla tightly and serve hot.

Chia Seed Pudding

Cook time: 8 hours (chilling time)

Serving: 1

Ingredients:

- 1/4 cup chia seeds
- 1 cup non-dairy milk (such as almond or coconut)
- 1 tablespoon honey or maple syrup
- 1/4 teaspoon vanilla extract
- Fresh berries for topping

Preparation:

1. In a mason jar or small bowl, mix together the chia seeds, non-dairy milk, honey or maple syrup, and vanilla extract.
2. Cover and refrigerate overnight or for at least 8 hours.
3. Before serving, top with fresh berries of your choice.

Avocado Toast with Poached Egg

Cook time: 10 minutes

Serving: 1

Ingredients:

- 1 slice whole grain bread, toasted
- 1/4 avocado, mashed
- 1 poached egg
- Salt and pepper to taste
- Lemon juice (optional)

Preparation:

1. In a small pot, bring a few inches of water to a simmer.
2. Crack an egg into a small bowl.
3. Using a spoon, create a whirlpool in the simmering water.
4. Gently pour the egg into the whirlpool and let cook for 3-4 minutes.
5. Use a slotted spoon to carefully remove the egg and place it on a paper towel to drain excess water.
6. Spread the mashed avocado on top of the toasted bread.
7. Place the poached egg on top of the avocado.
8. Sprinkle with salt and pepper, and squeeze a bit of lemon juice on top if desired.
9. Serve hot.

Smoothie Bowl with Almond Butter

Cook time: 5 minutes

Serving: 1

Ingredients:

- 1 ripe banana, frozen
- 1/2 cup frozen mixed berries
- 1/2 cup non-dairy milk (such as almond or coconut)
- 1 tablespoon almond butter

- 1 tablespoon toppings of your choice (such as granola, sliced fruit, or shredded coconut)

Preparation:
1. In a blender, add the frozen banana, frozen mixed berries, non-dairy milk, and almond butter.
2. Blend until smooth and creamy.
3. Pour the smoothie into a bowl.
4. Top with your choice of toppings.
5. Enjoy immediately.

Breakfast Quinoa Bowl

Cook time: 20 minutes

Serving: 2

Ingredients:
- 1/2 cup quinoa
- 1 cup water or vegetable broth
- 1/2 cup canned black beans, drained and rinsed
- 1/4 cup diced avocado
- 1/4 cup diced tomatoes
- 1/4 cup chopped bell peppers
- 2 tablespoons chopped cilantro
- Salt and pepper to taste
- Squeeze of lime juice (optional)

Preparation:
1. In a pot, bring the water or vegetable broth to a boil.
2. Add in the quinoa, reduce to a simmer, and cover.
3. Cook for 15 minutes until all the liquid is absorbed.
4. In a bowl, mix together the cooked quinoa, black beans, avocado, tomatoes, bell peppers, and cilantro.
5. Season with salt and pepper, and squeeze a bit of lime juice on top if desired.
6. Serve warm.

Chapter 2: Light and Filling Salads

Grilled Chicken Salad

Cook time: 20 minutes

Serving: 4

Ingredients:

- 1 lb chicken breast, sliced
- Salt and pepper to taste
- 1 tbsp olive oil
- 8 cups mixed greens
- 1 cup cherry tomatoes, halved
- 1 avocado, diced
- 1/4 cup red onion, thinly sliced
- 1/4 cup feta cheese, crumbled
- 1/4 cup balsamic vinaigrette dressing

Preparation:

1. Season the chicken breast with salt and pepper.
2. In a pan, heat olive oil over medium heat.
3. Add chicken to the pan and cook for 5-6 minutes on each side, until fully cooked.
4. Remove from heat and let it cool for a few minutes before slicing.
5. In a large bowl, add mixed greens, cherry tomatoes, avocado, red onion, and feta cheese.
6. Toss with balsamic vinaigrette dressing.
7. Top with sliced chicken and serve immediately.

Quinoa and Black Bean Salad

Cook time: 25 minutes

Serving: 4

Ingredients:

- 1 cup quinoa
- 2 cups water
- 1 can black beans, drained and rinsed
- 1 red bell pepper, diced
- 1/4 cup cilantro, chopped

- 1/4 cup red onion, diced
- 1 jalapeno, seeded and diced
- 1 avocado, diced
- Juice of 1 lime
- Salt and pepper to taste

Preparation:
1. In a pot, combine quinoa and water and bring to a boil.
2. Reduce heat to low and let it simmer for 15 minutes, until quinoa is fully cooked.
3. In a large bowl, combine cooked quinoa, black beans, red bell pepper, cilantro, red onion, jalapeno, avocado, and lime juice.
4. Season with salt and pepper.
5. Toss everything together until well combined.
6. Serve chilled or at room temperature.

Mediterranean Chickpea Salad

Cook time: 15 minutes

Serving: 4

Ingredients:
- 1 can chickpeas, drained and rinsed
- 1 cup cucumber, diced
- 1 cup cherry tomatoes, halved
- 1/2 cup Kalamata olives, sliced
- 1/4 cup red onion, diced
- 1/4 cup feta cheese, crumbled
- Juice of 1 lemon
- 2 tbsp olive oil
- 1 tsp dried oregano
- Salt and pepper to taste

Preparation:
1. In a large bowl, combine chickpeas, cucumber, cherry tomatoes, Kalamata olives, red onion, and feta cheese.
2. In a small bowl, whisk together lemon juice, olive oil, dried oregano, salt, and pepper.
3. Pour the dressing over the salad and mix well.

4. Serve immediately or refrigerate until ready to serve.

Spinach and Strawberry Salad

Cook time: 10 minutes

Serving: 4

Ingredients:

- 8 cups baby spinach
- 1 cup strawberries, sliced
- 1/4 cup red onion, thinly sliced
- 1/4 cup crumbled goat cheese
- 1/4 cup sliced almonds
- 1/4 cup balsamic vinaigrette dressing
- Salt and pepper to taste

Preparation:

1. In a large bowl, combine baby spinach, sliced strawberries, red onion, goat cheese, and sliced almonds.
2. Toss with balsamic vinaigrette dressing.
3. Season with salt and pepper to taste.
4. Serve immediately.

Thai Peanut Noodle Salad

Cook time: 15 minutes

Serving: 4

Ingredients:

- 8 oz rice noodles
- 1 red bell pepper, julienned
- 1 carrot, julienned
- 1/4 cup cilantro, chopped
- 1/4 cup green onions, sliced
- 1/4 cup chopped peanuts
- For the sauce:
- 1/4 cup creamy peanut butter
- 2 tbsp soy sauce
- 2 tbsp lime juice
- 1 tbsp honey

- 1 tsp sesame oil
- 1 tsp red pepper flakes (optional)
- Salt and pepper to taste

Preparation:
1. Bring a pot of water to a boil and cook rice noodles according to package instructions.
2. Drain and rinse noodles with cold water, set aside.
3. In a small bowl, whisk together peanut butter, soy sauce, lime juice, honey, sesame oil, red pepper flakes, salt, and pepper to make the sauce.
4. In a large bowl, combine cooked noodles, julienned bell pepper and carrot, chopped cilantro and green onions, and chopped peanuts.
5. Pour the prepared sauce over the noodle mixture and toss until well coated.
6. Serve immediately or refrigerate until ready to serve.

Roasted Vegetable Salad

Cook time: 30 minutes

Serving: 4

Ingredients:
- 1 red bell pepper, sliced
- 1 yellow bell pepper, sliced
- 1 zucchini, sliced
- 1 eggplant, sliced
- 1 red onion, sliced
- 4 cups arugula
- 1/4 cup crumbled goat cheese
- 1/4 cup chopped walnuts
- Balsamic vinaigrette (or dressing of your choice)

Preparation:
1. Preheat your oven to 400 degrees F (200 degrees C).
2. In a large baking dish, toss the sliced red and yellow bell peppers, zucchini, eggplant, and red onion with olive oil, salt, and pepper.
3. Roast for 20-25 minutes, stirring halfway.
4. Allow the roasted vegetables to cool for a few minutes.

5. Place arugula on a large serving platter and top with the roasted vegetables.
6. Sprinkle crumbled goat cheese and chopped walnuts over the vegetables.
7. Drizzle with balsamic vinaigrette (or dressing of your choice).
8. Serve and enjoy!

Cobb Salad

Cook time: 20 minutes

Serving: 4

Ingredients:

- 6 cups chopped romaine lettuce
- 4 hard-boiled eggs, chopped
- 8 slices cooked bacon, chopped
- 1 cup cherry tomatoes, halved
- 1 avocado, chopped
- 1/2 cup crumbled blue cheese
- 2 grilled chicken breasts, chopped
- Ranch dressing (or dressing of your choice)

Preparation:

1. In a large bowl, combine chopped romaine lettuce, hard-boiled eggs, cooked bacon, cherry tomatoes, avocado, and crumbled blue cheese.
2. Top with chopped grilled chicken.
3. Drizzle with ranch dressing (or dressing of your choice).
4. Toss to combine and serve.

Tuna Salad Lettuce Wraps

Cook time: 10 minutes

Serving: 4

Ingredients:

- 2 cans of tuna, drained and flaked
- 1/4 cup diced red onion
- 1/4 cup diced celery
- 1/4 cup diced red bell pepper
- 1/4 cup diced carrots
- 1/4 cup mayonnaise

- 1 tsp dijon mustard
- Salt and pepper to taste
- 8 large lettuce leaves (such as romaine or butter lettuce)

Preparation:
1. In a bowl, mix together the tuna, red onion, celery, red bell pepper, and carrots.
2. In a separate small bowl, whisk together the mayonnaise, dijon mustard, salt, and pepper.
3. Pour the dressing over the tuna mixture and stir to combine.
4. Spoon the tuna salad onto the lettuce leaves.
5. Roll up the lettuce leaves to create a wrap.
6. Serve and enjoy!

Caprese Salad

Cook time: 5 minutes

Serving: 4

Ingredients:
- 2 large beefsteak tomatoes, sliced
- 8 oz fresh mozzarella, sliced
- 1/4 cup balsamic vinegar
- 1/4 cup extra virgin olive oil
- Salt and pepper to taste
- Fresh basil leaves

Preparation:
1. On a large platter, arrange the tomato and mozzarella slices alternately.
2. In a small bowl, whisk together balsamic vinegar, olive oil, salt, and pepper.
3. Drizzle the dressing over the tomato and mozzarella slices.
4. Top with fresh basil leaves.
5. Serve and enjoy!

Watermelon and Feta Salad

Cook time: 10 minutes

Serving: 4

Ingredients:

- 4 cups cubed watermelon
- 1/2 cup crumbled feta cheese
- 1/4 cup chopped fresh mint
- 1/4 cup chopped fresh basil
- 1/4 cup chopped red onion
- 2 tbsp olive oil
- 1 tbsp balsamic vinegar
- Salt and pepper to taste

Preparation:
1. In a large bowl, combine watermelon, feta cheese, mint, basil, and red onion.
2. In a separate small bowl, whisk together olive oil, balsamic vinegar, salt, and pepper.
3. Pour the dressing over the watermelon mixture and toss to combine.
4. Serve and enjoy!

Chapter 3: Hearty Soups

Minestrone Soup

Cook time: 45 minutes

Serving: 4-6

Ingredients:
- 1 tbsp olive oil
- 1 onion, diced
- 3 cloves of garlic, minced
- 2 stalks of celery, diced
- 1 carrot, diced
- 1 zucchini, diced
- 1 can of diced tomatoes (14.5 oz)
- 4 cups of vegetable broth
- 1 can of kidney beans, rinsed and drained (14.5 oz)
- 1 cup of small pasta, such as elbow or ditalini
- 1 tsp dried oregano

- 1 tsp dried basil
- Salt and pepper to taste
- Grated Parmesan cheese (optional)

Preparation:
1. Heat olive oil in a large pot over medium heat.
2. Add onions and garlic and cook until fragrant, about 2-3 minutes.
3. Add celery, carrots, and zucchini and cook for an additional 5 minutes.
4. Pour in diced tomatoes and vegetable broth and bring to a boil.
5. Reduce heat and let simmer for 25 minutes.
6. Add kidney beans, pasta, oregano, and basil to the pot and let cook for 10 minutes or until pasta is al dente.
7. Season with salt and pepper to taste.
8. Serve hot and top with grated Parmesan cheese, if desired.

Lentil Soup

Cook time: 30 minutes

Serving: 4-6

Ingredients:
- 1 tbsp olive oil
- 1 onion, diced
- 3 cloves of garlic, minced
- 1 carrot, diced
- 1 celery stick, diced
- 2 potatoes, peeled and diced
- 1 cup of dried lentils, rinsed and drained
- 4 cups of vegetable broth
- 1 bay leaf
- 1 tsp dried thyme
- Salt and pepper to taste
- Parsley for garnish (optional)

Preparation:
1. Heat olive oil in a large pot over medium heat.
2. Add onions and garlic and cook until fragrant, about 2-3 minutes.
3. Add carrots, celery, and potatoes and cook for an additional 5 minutes.
4. Stir in lentils, vegetable broth, bay leaf, and thyme.

5. Bring to a boil, then reduce heat and let simmer for 20 minutes or until lentils are tender.
6. Season with salt and pepper to taste.
7. Remove bay leaf before serving.
8. Optional: Garnish with chopped parsley before serving.

Chicken and Vegetable Soup

Cook time: 45 minutes

Serving: 4-6

Ingredients:

- 1 tbsp olive oil
- 1 onion, diced
- 3 cloves of garlic, minced
- 2 carrots, peeled and diced
- 1 celery stalk, diced
- 1 red bell pepper, diced
- 6 cups of chicken broth
- 1 cup of diced cooked chicken
- 1 cup of frozen corn
- 1 cup of frozen peas
- 1 tsp dried thyme
- 1 tsp dried oregano
- Salt and pepper to taste
- Fresh parsley for garnish (optional)

Preparation:

1. Heat olive oil in a large pot over medium heat.
2. Add onions and garlic and cook until fragrant, about 2-3 minutes.
3. Add carrots, celery, and bell pepper and cook for an additional 5 minutes.
4. Pour in chicken broth and bring to a boil.
5. Add diced chicken, corn, peas, thyme, and oregano.
6. Let simmer for 20 minutes.
7. Season with salt and pepper to taste.
8. Optional: Garnish with fresh parsley before serving.

Butternut Squash Soup

Cook time: 40 minutes

Serving: 4-6

Ingredients:

- 2 tbsp butter
- 1 onion, diced
- 3 cloves of garlic, minced
- 1 butternut squash, peeled and diced
- 2 potatoes, peeled and diced
- 4 cups of vegetable broth
- 1 tsp dried thyme
- 1 tsp dried sage
- Salt and pepper to taste
- Pumpkin seeds for garnish (optional)

Preparation:

1. In a large pot, melt butter over medium heat.
2. Add onions and garlic and cook until fragrant, 2-3 minutes.
3. Add butternut squash and potatoes and cook for an additional 5 minutes.
4. Pour in vegetable broth and bring to a boil.
5. Let simmer for 25 minutes or until vegetables are tender.
6. Using an immersion blender, puree the soup until smooth.
7. Stir in thyme and sage.
8. Season with salt and pepper to taste.
9. Optional: Garnish with pumpkin seeds before serving.

Gazpacho

Cook time: 10 minutes

Serving: 4-6

Ingredients:

- 4 cups of tomatoes, diced
- 1 cucumber, peeled and diced
- 1 red bell pepper, diced
- 1 small onion, diced
- 3 cloves of garlic, minced
- 3 tbsp red wine vinegar
- 2 tbsp olive oil

- 1 tsp dried oregano
- 1 tsp dried basil
- Salt and pepper to taste
- Croutons for garnish (optional)

Preparation:
1. In a blender or food processor, combine tomatoes, cucumber, red bell pepper, onion, garlic, red wine vinegar, olive oil, oregano, and basil.
2. Blend until smooth.
3. Season with salt and pepper to taste.
4. Refrigerate for at least 1 hour before serving.
5. Optional: Serve with croutons on top for added texture and flavor.

Tom Yum Soup

Cook time: 30 minutes

Serving: 4-6

Ingredients:
- 4 cups of vegetable or chicken broth
- 1 stalk of lemongrass, smashed
- 2 inches of galangal, peeled and sliced
- 3 kaffir lime leaves
- 3 cloves of garlic, minced
- 2 red chili peppers, diced
- 1 cup of button mushrooms, sliced
- 1 tomato, diced
- 1 cup of diced tofu
- 1 tbsp fish sauce
- 1 tbsp soy sauce
- 1 tbsp lime juice
- Cilantro for garnish (optional)

Preparation:
1. In a pot, bring vegetable or chicken broth to a boil.
2. Add lemongrass, galangal, kaffir lime leaves, garlic, and chili peppers.
3. Let simmer for 15 minutes.
4. Add mushrooms, tomato, tofu, fish sauce, soy sauce, and lime juice.
5. Simmer for an additional 10 minutes.

6. Remove lemongrass stalk and kaffir lime leaves before serving.

7. Optional: Garnish with cilantro before serving.

Split Pea Soup

Cook time: 1 hour

Serving: 4-6

Ingredients:

- 1 tbsp olive oil
- 1 onion, diced
- 3 cloves of garlic, minced
- 2 carrots, peeled and diced
- 2 celery stalks, diced
- 2 cups of split peas, rinsed and drained
- 6 cups of vegetable or chicken broth
- 1 tsp dried thyme
- 1 tsp smoked paprika
- Salt and pepper to taste
- Crumbled bacon for garnish (optional)

Preparation:

1. Heat olive oil in a pot over medium heat.
2. Add onions and garlic and cook until fragrant, 2-3 minutes.
3. Add carrots and celery and cook for an additional 5 minutes.
4. Stir in split peas and broth.
5. Bring to a boil, then reduce heat and let simmer for 45 minutes to 1 hour, until peas are tender.
6. Stir in thyme and smoked paprika.
7. Season with salt and pepper to taste.
8. Optional: Serve with crumbled bacon on top for added flavor.

Turkey Chili

Cook time: 40 minutes

Serving: 4-6

Ingredients:

- 1 tbsp olive oil
- 1 onion, diced

- 3 cloves of garlic, minced
- 2 lbs ground turkey
- 1 red bell pepper, diced
- 1 can of kidney beans, rinsed and drained (14.5 oz)
- 1 can of black beans, rinsed and drained (14.5 oz)
- 1 can of diced tomatoes (14.5 oz)
- 1 cup of chicken broth
- 2 tbsp chili powder
- 1 tsp cumin
- 1 tsp dried oregano
- Salt and pepper to taste
- Shredded cheddar cheese for garnish (optional)

Preparation:
1. Heat olive oil in a large pot over medium heat.
2. Add onions and garlic and cook until fragrant, 2-3 minutes.
3. Add ground turkey and cook until browned.
4. Stir in bell pepper and cook for an additional 5 minutes.
5. Add kidney beans, black beans, diced tomatoes, chicken broth, chili powder, cumin, and oregano.
6. Bring to a boil, then reduce heat and let simmer for 20 minutes.
7. Season with salt and pepper to taste.
8. Optional: Serve with shredded cheddar cheese on top for added flavor.

Creamy Broccoli Soup

Cook time: 30 minutes

Serving: 4-6

Ingredients:
- 2 tbsp butter
- 1 onion, diced
- 3 cloves of garlic, minced
- 6 cups of broccoli florets
- 4 cups of chicken or vegetable broth
- 1 cup of heavy cream
- 1 cup of shredded cheddar cheese
- Salt and pepper to taste
- Croutons for garnish (optional)

Preparation:

1. In a large pot, melt butter over medium heat.
2. Add onions and garlic and cook until fragrant, 2-3 minutes.
3. Add broccoli florets and cook for an additional 5 minutes.
4. Pour in chicken or vegetable broth and bring to a boil.
5. Reduce heat and let simmer for 15 minutes.
6. Using an immersion blender, puree the soup until smooth.
7. Stir in heavy cream and cheddar cheese until cheese is melted.
8. Season with salt and pepper to taste.
9. Optional: Serve with croutons on top for added texture.

Mushroom Barley Soup

Cook time: 1 hour

Serving: 4-6

Ingredients:

- 2 tbsp olive oil
- 1 onion, diced
- 3 cloves of garlic, minced
- 8 oz white mushrooms, sliced
- 8 oz cremini mushrooms, sliced
- 6 cups of beef or vegetable broth
- 1 cup of pearl barley
- 1 tsp dried thyme
- 1 tsp dried parsley
- Salt and pepper to taste
- Fresh parsley for garnish (optional)

Preparation:

1. Heat olive oil in a pot over medium heat.
2. Add onions and garlic and cook until fragrant, 2-3 minutes.
3. Stir in mushrooms and cook until softened.
4. Pour in broth and bring to a boil.
5. Add pearl barley and reduce heat to low.
6. Let simmer for 45 minutes to 1 hour, until barley is tender.
7. Stir in thyme and parsley.
8. Season with salt and pepper to taste.

9.   Optional: Garnish with fresh parsley before serving.

Chapter 4: Lean Proteins

Baked Salmon with Lemon-Dill Sauce

Cook time: 20 minutes

Serves: 4

Ingredients:

- 4 salmon fillets (6 oz each)
- Salt and pepper
- 3 tbsp olive oil
- 2 tbsp lemon juice
- 2 cloves of garlic, minced
- 1 tsp dried dill
- 1/4 cup mayonnaise
- 1/4 cup plain Greek yogurt
- Lemon wedges, for serving

Preparation:

1.   Preheat your oven to 375°F (190°C).
2.   Season the salmon fillets with salt and pepper on both sides.
3.   In a small bowl, mix together the olive oil, lemon juice, minced garlic, and dried dill. Brush this mixture over the salmon fillets.
4.   Place the salmon fillets on a baking dish and bake for 15-18 minutes, or until they are cooked through.
5.   While the salmon is baking, make the lemon-dill sauce. In a small bowl, mix together the mayonnaise, Greek yogurt, lemon juice, and dried dill.
6.   Serve the baked salmon with the lemon-dill sauce on top and lemon wedges on the side. Enjoy!

Grilled Shrimp Skewers

Cook time: 15 minutes

Serves: 4

Ingredients:

- 1 lb shrimp, peeled and deveined
- 2 tbsp olive oil
- 2 cloves of garlic, minced
- 1 tsp paprika
- 1 tsp Italian seasoning
- Salt and pepper
- Wooden or metal skewers
- Lemon wedges and parsley, for serving

Preparation:

1. If using wooden skewers, soak them in water for 30 minutes before grilling to prevent burning.
2. In a large bowl, mix together the olive oil, minced garlic, paprika, Italian seasoning, salt, and pepper.
3. Add the shrimp to the bowl and toss to coat them in the marinade.
4. Thread the shrimp onto the skewers.
5. Heat a grill or grill pan over medium high heat. Place the skewers on the grill and cook for 3-4 minutes on each side, or until the shrimp are pink and cooked through.
6. Serve the grilled shrimp skewers with lemon wedges and fresh parsley on top. Enjoy!

Turkey Meatballs

Cook time: 25 minutes

Serves: 4

Ingredients:

- 1 lb ground turkey
- 1/2 cup breadcrumbs
- 1/4 cup grated parmesan cheese
- 2 cloves of garlic, minced
- 1/4 cup chopped fresh parsley
- 1 egg
- Salt and pepper
- Marinara sauce, for serving

Preparation:

1. Preheat your oven to 375°F (190°C).

2. In a large bowl, mix together the ground turkey, breadcrumbs, parmesan cheese, minced garlic, chopped parsley, egg, salt, and pepper.
3. Roll the mixture into 1-inch meatballs and place them on a baking sheet lined with parchment paper.
4. Bake the meatballs for 20-25 minutes, or until they are cooked through.
5. Serve the turkey meatballs with your favorite marinara sauce. Enjoy!

Tofu Stir-Fry

Cook time: 20 minutes

Serves: 4

Ingredients:

- 1 block extra firm tofu, drained and cubed
- 2 tbsp soy sauce
- 2 tbsp sesame oil
- 2 tbsp honey
- 1 tbsp rice vinegar
- 1 tbsp cornstarch
- 1 tbsp water
- 1 tbsp vegetable oil
- 2 cloves of garlic, minced
- 1 inch fresh ginger, minced
- 1 red bell pepper, sliced
- 1 cup broccoli florets
- 1 carrot, sliced
- 1 cup mushrooms, sliced
- Cooked rice, for serving

Preparation:

1. Mix together the soy sauce, sesame oil, honey, and rice vinegar in a small bowl.
2. In a separate small bowl, mix together the cornstarch and water to create a slurry.
3. Heat the vegetable oil in a large pan or wok over medium high heat.
4. Add the cubed tofu to the pan and cook for 2-3 minutes on each side, or until it starts to brown.
5. Remove the tofu from the pan and set aside.
6. In the same pan, add the minced garlic and ginger and stir fry for 1 minute.

7. Add the red bell pepper, broccoli, carrot, and mushrooms to the pan and stir fry for 3-4 minutes, or until the vegetables are tender.
8. Add the cooked tofu back into the pan.
9. Pour the soy sauce mixture over the tofu and vegetables, then add the cornstarch slurry.
10. Stir everything together and cook for an additional 2-3 minutes, or until the sauce thickens.
11. Serve the tofu stir-fry over cooked rice. Enjoy!

Baked Cod with Herbs

Cook time: 15 minutes

Serves: 4

Ingredients:
- 4 cod fillets (6 oz each)
- Salt and pepper
- 2 tbsp olive oil
- 2 cloves of garlic, minced
- 1 tsp dried thyme
- 1 tsp dried oregano
- 1 tbsp lemon juice
- Lemon wedges, for serving

Preparation:
1. Preheat your oven to 375°F (190°C).
2. Season the cod fillets with salt and pepper.
3. In a small bowl, mix together the olive oil, minced garlic, dried thyme, dried oregano, and lemon juice.
4. Brush the herb mixture over the cod fillets.
5. Place the fillets on a baking dish and bake for 12-15 minutes, or until they are cooked through and flaky.
6. Serve the baked cod with lemon wedges on the side. Enjoy!

Pork Tenderloin with Apple Chutney

Cook time: 40 minutes

Serving: 4-6

Ingredients:

- 1 pork tenderloin (about 1.5 lbs)
- 2 tbsp olive oil
- 1 tsp salt
- 1 tsp black pepper
- 1/2 tsp garlic powder
- 1/2 tsp dried thyme
- 2 tbsp butter
- 2 apples, peeled and diced
- 1/2 cup diced onion
- 1/4 cup brown sugar
- 1/4 cup apple cider vinegar
- 1/4 tsp ground cinnamon
- 1/4 tsp ground ginger
- 1/4 cup water

Preparation:

1. Preheat your oven to 375°F (190°C).
2. In a small bowl, mix together 1 tbsp of olive oil, salt, black pepper, garlic powder, and dried thyme to create a rub for the pork tenderloin.
3. Rub the seasoning mixture all over the pork tenderloin.
4. Heat the remaining olive oil in a large skillet over medium-high heat. Sear the pork tenderloin on all sides until browned, about 2 minutes per side.
5. Transfer the pork tenderloin to a baking dish and bake for 25-30 minutes, or until the internal temperature reaches 145°F (63°C).
6. While the pork is cooking, prepare the apple chutney. In the same skillet used for the pork, melt the butter over medium heat. Add in the diced apples and onions and cook until both are softened, about 5 minutes.
7. Add in the brown sugar, apple cider vinegar, cinnamon, ginger, and water. Stir to combine.
8. Let the chutney simmer for about 10 minutes, until it thickens and the apples are cooked through.
9. Once the pork is fully cooked, let it rest for 5 minutes before slicing.
10. Serve the sliced pork with the apple chutney on top. Enjoy!

Lemon Herb Grilled Chicken

Cook time: 20 minutes

Serving: 4-6

Ingredients:

- 4-6 chicken breasts
- 1/4 cup olive oil
- Juice of 1 lemon
- 2 garlic cloves, minced
- 1 tsp dried oregano
- 1 tsp dried thyme
- 1 tsp dried rosemary
- 1 tsp salt
- 1/2 tsp black pepper

Preparation:

1. In a large bowl, whisk together the olive oil, lemon juice, minced garlic, dried oregano, dried thyme, dried rosemary, salt, and black pepper.
2. Add the chicken breasts to the bowl and coat them in the marinade. Cover and let marinate in the fridge for at least 30 minutes, or up to 2 hours.
3. Preheat your grill to medium-high heat.
4. Grill the chicken for about 5-7 minutes per side, or until fully cooked and the internal temperature reaches 165°F (74°C).
5. Let the chicken rest for 5 minutes before slicing. Serve and enjoy!

Beef and Broccoli Stir-Fry

Cook time: 20 minutes

Serving: 4

Ingredients:

- 1 lb flank steak, sliced against the grain
- 2 tbsp olive oil
- 2 cloves garlic, minced
- 1 inch ginger, minced
- 1/2 onion, sliced
- 2 cups broccoli florets
- 1 red bell pepper, sliced
- 1/4 cup low-sodium soy sauce
- 2 tbsp brown sugar
- 1 tbsp cornstarch
- 1/4 cup water
- Cooked rice, for serving

Preparation:

1. In a large skillet or wok, heat the olive oil over high heat.
2. Add the sliced flank steak to the skillet and cook for about 3-4 minutes, or until browned.
3. Add in the minced garlic and ginger and cook for another 2 minutes.
4. Next, add in the sliced onion, broccoli florets, and red bell pepper. Stir-fry for 5-7 minutes, until the vegetables are cooked but still crisp.
5. In a small bowl, mix together the soy sauce, brown sugar, cornstarch, and water. Pour the sauce over the beef and vegetables.
6. Let the stir-fry cook for an additional 2-3 minutes, until the sauce has thickened and coats the beef and vegetables.
7. Serve over cooked rice and enjoy!

Vegetarian Chili

Cook time: 45 minutes

Serving: 6-8

Ingredients:

- 1 tbsp olive oil
- 1 onion, diced
- 3 cloves garlic, minced
- 2 carrots, diced
- 1 red bell pepper, diced
- 1 jalapeno, seeds removed and diced
- 2 tsp chili powder
- 1 tsp cumin
- 1 tsp smoked paprika
- 1/4 tsp cayenne pepper
- 1 can (28 oz) diced tomatoes
- 1 can (15 oz) black beans, drained and rinsed
- 1 can (15 oz) kidney beans, drained and rinsed
- 1 cup vegetable broth
- Salt and pepper, to taste
- Optional toppings: shredded cheese, sour cream, diced avocado, chopped cilantro

Preparation:

1. In a large pot, heat the olive oil over medium heat.
2. Add in the diced onion, minced garlic, diced carrots, diced red bell pepper, and diced jalapeno. Cook for about 5 minutes, until the vegetables are softened.
3. Stir in the chili powder, cumin, smoked paprika, and cayenne pepper. Cook for an additional 2 minutes.
4. Pour in the diced tomatoes, black beans, kidney beans, and vegetable broth. Stir to combine.
5. Bring the chili to a boil, then reduce the heat to low and let it simmer for 30 minutes.
6. Season with salt and pepper, to taste.
7. Serve the chili hot with your desired toppings. Enjoy!

Teriyaki Tempeh

Cook time: 20 minutes

Serving: 4

Ingredients:

- 8 oz tempeh, sliced into 1/2 inch pieces
- 1/4 cup low-sodium soy sauce
- 1 tbsp honey
- 1 tbsp rice vinegar
- 1 tsp minced ginger
- 2 cloves garlic, minced
- 2 tbsp olive oil
- Cooked rice, for serving
- Optional toppings: sliced green onions, sesame seeds

Preparation:

1. In a shallow dish, mix together the soy sauce, honey, rice vinegar, minced ginger, and minced garlic.
2. Add the sliced tempeh to the marinade and let it marinate for at least 10 minutes.
3. Heat the olive oil in a large skillet over medium-high heat.
4. Add the marinated tempeh to the skillet and cook for 3-4 minutes on each side, until browned.

5. Pour the remaining marinade over the tempeh in the skillet and let it cook for an additional 2-3 minutes, until the sauce thickens and coats the tempeh.
6. Serve the teriyaki tempeh over cooked rice and top with sliced green onions and sesame seeds, if desired. Enjoy!

Chapter 5: Wholesome Sides

Roasted Brussels Sprouts

Cook time: 25 minutes

Serving: 4

Ingredients:

- 1 pound Brussels sprouts, trimmed and halved
- 2 tablespoons olive oil
- 2 cloves garlic, minced
- 1 teaspoon salt
- 1/2 teaspoon black pepper
- 1/4 cup grated Parmesan cheese

Preparation:
1. Preheat the oven to 400°F (200°C).
2. In a large bowl, toss Brussels sprouts with olive oil, garlic, salt, and pepper.
3. Spread the Brussels sprouts in a single layer on a baking sheet.
4. Roast in the preheated oven for 20-25 minutes, stirring occasionally, until lightly browned and tender.
5. Sprinkle with grated Parmesan cheese before serving.

Quinoa Pilaf

Cook time: 25 minutes

Serving: 4

Ingredients:

- 1 cup quinoa, rinsed and drained

- 2 cups water or vegetable broth
- 1 tablespoon olive oil
- 1 onion, diced
- 2 cloves garlic, minced
- 1 red bell pepper, diced
- 1 cup frozen peas
- 1/4 cup chopped parsley
- Salt and pepper to taste

Preparation:

1. In a medium pot, bring the water or vegetable broth to a boil. Add quinoa, reduce heat to low, cover, and simmer for 15 minutes.
2. In a separate pan, heat olive oil over medium heat. Add onion and garlic and cook until softened, about 5 minutes.
3. Add the diced bell pepper and frozen peas to the pan and cook for an additional 5 minutes.
4. Add the cooked quinoa to the pan with the vegetables and stir to combine.
5. Season with salt, pepper, and parsley before serving.

Garlic Roasted Asparagus

Cook time: 15 minutes

Serving: 4

Ingredients:

- 1-pound asparagus, trimmed
- 2 tablespoons olive oil
- 3 cloves garlic, minced
- Salt and pepper to taste

Preparation:

1. Preheat the oven to 425°F (220°C).
2. In a large bowl, toss asparagus with olive oil, garlic, salt, and pepper.
3. Spread the asparagus in a single layer on a baking sheet.
4. Roast in the preheated oven for 12-15 minutes, or until tender.
5. Serve as a side dish or sprinkle with Parmesan cheese before serving.

Sweet Potato Fries

Cook time: 30 minutes

Serving: 4

Ingredients:

- 2 large sweet potatoes, peeled and cut into fries
- 2 tablespoons olive oil
- 1 tablespooncornstarch
- 1 teaspoon garlic powder
- 1 teaspoon paprika
- Salt and pepper to taste

Preparation:

1. Preheat the oven to 425°F (220°C).
2. In a large bowl, toss sweet potato fries with olive oil, cornstarch, garlic powder, paprika, salt, and pepper.
3. Spread the fries in a single layer on a baking sheet.
4. Bake for 30 minutes, turning halfway through, until crispy and golden brown.
5. Serve as a delicious and healthier alternative to traditional fries.

Steamed Broccoli with Lemon

Cook time: 10 minutes

Serving: 4

Ingredients:

- 1 head of broccoli, cut into florets
- 1 tablespoon olive oil
- 1 tablespoon lemon juice
- Salt and pepper to taste

Preparation:

1. In a large pot, bring 1 inch of water to a boil.
2. Place a steamer basket or colander over the pot, making sure it does not touch the water.
3. Add the broccoli florets to the steamer basket and cover with a lid.
4. Steam for 5-7 minutes, or until broccoli is tender.
5. In a small bowl, mix together olive oil, lemon juice, salt, and pepper.
6. Drizzle the dressing over the steamed broccoli before serving.

Cauliflower Mash

Cook time: 20 minutes

Serving: 4

Ingredients:

- 1 head of cauliflower, chopped into florets
- 2 tablespoons butter
- 2 cloves garlic, minced
- 1/4 cup milk (or non-dairy alternative)
- Salt and pepper to taste

Preparation:

1. In a large pot, bring water to a boil. Add the cauliflower florets and cook for 10-12 minutes, or until tender.
2. Drain the cauliflower and place in a food processor.
3. In a small pan, melt butter over medium heat. Add minced garlic and cook for 1-2 minutes.
4. Add the garlic butter and milk to the food processor with the cauliflower. Blend until smooth.
5. Season with salt and pepper before serving.

Cucumber Salad

Cook time: 10 minutes

Serving: 4

Ingredients:

- 1 large English cucumber, thinly sliced
- 1/4 cup red onion, thinly sliced
- 1/4 cup white vinegar
- 1 tablespoon sugar
- Salt and pepper to taste

Preparation:

1. In a large bowl, combine sliced cucumber and onion.
2. In a small bowl, mix together vinegar, sugar, salt, and pepper.
3. Pour the vinegar mixture over the cucumber and onion, tossing to coat.
4. Let the salad marinate in the fridge for at least 30 minutes before serving.

Roasted Beets with Goat Cheese

Cook time: 45 minutes

Serving: 4

Ingredients:

- 4 beets, peeled and cut into wedges
- 2 tablespoons olive oil
- 2 tablespoons balsamic vinegar
- Salt and pepper to taste
- 4 ounces' goat cheese, crumbled

Preparation:

1. Preheat the oven to 400°F (200°C).
2. In a large bowl, toss beet wedges with olive oil, balsamic vinegar, salt, and pepper.
3. Spread the beets in a single layer on a baking sheet.
4. Roast for 35-40 minutes, or until tender.
5. Sprinkle crumbled goat cheese over the roasted beets before serving.

Sauteed Spinach with Garlic

Cook time: 10 minutes

Serving: 4

Ingredients:

- 2 tablespoons olive oil
- 2 cloves garlic, minced
- 10 oz fresh spinach
- Salt and pepper to taste

Preparation:

1. In a large pan, heat olive oil over medium heat.
2. Add minced garlic and cook for 1-2 minutes.
3. Add the spinach and sauté for 3-5 minutes, or until wilted.
4. Season with salt and pepper before serving.

Grilled Corn on the Cob

Cook time: 20 minutes

Serving: 4

Ingredients:

- 4 ears of corn, husks removed
- 2 tablespoons butter
- Salt and pepper to taste

Preparation:

1. Preheat the grill to medium heat.
2. Place corn on the grill and cook for 10 minutes, turning occasionally.
3. Melt butter in the microwave or on the stovetop.
4. Brush butter over the corn and continue grilling for 5-7 minutes, or until tender.
5. Season with salt and pepper before serving.

Chapter 6: Vegetarian Delights

Eggplant Parmesan

Cook time: 1 hour

Serving: 4

Ingredients:

- 1 large eggplant, sliced into 1/2 inch rounds
- 1 cup flour
- 2 eggs, beaten
- 1 cup Italian seasoned breadcrumbs
- 1 cup marinara sauce
- 1 cup shredded mozzarella cheese
- 1/4 cup grated parmesan cheese
- 1 tablespoon olive oil
- Salt and pepper to taste

Preparation:

1. Preheat your oven to 375°F (190°C).
2. Season the eggplant slices with salt and pepper on both sides.
3. Dip the eggplant slices in flour, then in beaten eggs, and finally in breadcrumbs, making sure to coat them evenly.
4. Heat olive oil in a large skillet over medium heat and cook the eggplant slices for about 2-3 minutes on each side, until they are lightly browned.
5. In a greased 9x13 inch baking dish, spread a thin layer of marinara sauce on the bottom.
6. Arrange the cooked eggplant slices in a single layer over the marinara sauce.
7. Spread another layer of marinara sauce over the eggplant slices and sprinkle with both mozzarella and parmesan cheese.
8. Repeat layers until all eggplant slices are used, and make sure to end with a layer of sauce and cheese on top.
9. Bake in the preheated oven for 35-40 minutes, until the cheese is golden and bubbly.
10. Let it cool for a few minutes before serving. Enjoy your delicious eggplant parmesan!

Spinach and Mushroom Stuffed Bell Peppers

Cook time: 45 minutes

Serving: 4

Ingredients:

- 4 bell peppers, sliced in half and seeds removed
- 1 cup cooked quinoa
- 1 cup diced mushrooms
- 1 cup chopped spinach
- 1 small onion, diced
- 2 cloves garlic, minced
- 1/2 cup shredded mozzarella cheese
- 1/4 cup grated parmesan cheese
- 1 tablespoon olive oil
- Salt and pepper to taste

Preparation:

1. Preheat your oven to 375°F (190°C).

2. In a large skillet, heat olive oil over medium heat. Sauté the onions and garlic until they are soft and fragrant, about 2-3 minutes.
3. Add diced mushrooms and chopped spinach to the skillet and cook until they are slightly wilted, about 2-3 minutes.
4. Stir in the cooked quinoa and season with salt and pepper.
5. Slice the bell peppers in half and remove the seeds. Place them in a greased baking dish.
6. Stuff the bell peppers with the quinoa and vegetable mixture.
7. Top each pepper with shredded mozzarella and grated parmesan cheese.
8. Bake in the preheated oven for 25-30 minutes until the peppers are tender and the cheese is melted and golden brown.
9. Let them cool for a few minutes before serving. Enjoy your delicious spinach and mushroom stuffed bell peppers!

Lentil and Vegetable Stir-Fry

Cook time: 45 minutes

Serving: 4

Ingredients:

- 1 cup dried lentils
- 1 cup diced bell peppers
- 1 cup diced carrots
- 1 cup chopped broccoli
- 1/2 cup sliced mushrooms
- 1 small onion, diced
- 2 cloves garlic, minced
- 1/4 cup low-sodium soy sauce
- 2 tablespoons sesame oil
- Salt and pepper to taste
- Cooked rice for serving

Preparation:

1. Cook lentils according to package instructions.
2. In a large skillet or wok, heat sesame oil over medium-high heat.
3. Add onions and garlic to the skillet and cook for 2-3 minutes until they are soft and fragrant.

4. Add diced bell peppers, carrots, broccoli, and mushrooms to the skillet and cook until they are slightly softened.
5. Stir in cooked lentils and season with salt and pepper.
6. Pour in low-sodium soy sauce and stir-fry for another 2-3 minutes.
7. Serve over cooked rice and enjoy your delicious lentil and vegetable stir-fry!

Chickpea Curry

Cook time: 40 minutes

Serving: 4

Ingredients:

- 1 can chickpeas, drained and rinsed
- 1 cup diced potatoes
- 1/2 cup diced carrots
- 1 small onion, diced
- 2 cloves garlic, minced
- 1 cup canned diced tomatoes
- 1 cup vegetable broth
- 2 tablespoons curry powder
- 1 tablespoon olive oil
- Salt and pepper to taste
- Cooked rice for serving

Preparation:

1. In a large pot, heat olive oil over medium heat. Sauté onions and garlic until they are soft and fragrant, about 2-3 minutes.
2. Add diced potatoes and carrots to the pot and cook for another 2-3 minutes.
3. Pour in canned diced tomatoes and vegetable broth. Season with salt, pepper, and curry powder.
4. Stir in chickpeas and let it simmer for 25-30 minutes until potatoes and carrots are tender.
5. Serve over cooked rice and enjoy your delicious chickpea curry!

Zucchini Noodles with Pesto

Cook time: 20 minutes

Serving: 2

Ingredients:

- 3 large zucchinis, spiralized into noodles
- 1 cup fresh basil leaves
- 1/4 cup pine nuts
- 1/4 cup grated parmesan cheese
- 2 cloves garlic, minced
- 1/4 cup olive oil
- Salt and pepper to taste
- Optional toppings: cherry tomatoes, diced bell peppers, chopped fresh herbs

Preparation:

1. In a food processor, blend together basil leaves, pine nuts, parmesan cheese, and garlic until smooth.
2. Slowly add in olive oil and continue blending until a smooth pesto sauce forms. Season with salt and pepper to taste.
3. In a large skillet, heat olive oil over medium heat. Add zucchini noodles and cook for 2-3 minutes until they are tender.
4. Pour in the pesto sauce and stir until noodles are evenly coated.
5. Optional: top with cherry tomatoes, diced bell peppers, or chopped fresh herbs before serving. Enjoy your delicious zucchini noodles with pesto!

Black Bean Tacos

Cook time: 20 minutes

Serving: 4

Ingredients:

- 1 can black beans, drained and rinsed
- 1 bell pepper, diced
- 1 onion, diced
- 1 tsp cumin
- 1 tsp chili powder
- Salt and pepper to taste
- Tortillas
- Toppings of choice (avocado, salsa, cilantro, etc.)

Preparation:

1. In a pan over medium heat, sauté bell pepper and onion until softened.

2. Add black beans, cumin, chili powder, and salt and pepper to the pan with the vegetables. Cook for 5 minutes.
3. Warm tortillas in another pan over low heat.
4. Fill tortillas with the black bean mixture and top with desired toppings.
5. Serve and enjoy.

Vegan Chili

Cook time: 45 minutes

Serving: 6

Ingredients:

- 1 onion, diced
- 2 cloves garlic, minced
- 1 can diced tomatoes
- 1 can kidney beans, drained and rinsed
- 1 can black beans, drained and rinsed
- 1 can corn, drained
- 2 tbsp chili powder
- 1 tsp cumin
- 1 tsp paprika
- 1 tsp oregano
- Salt and pepper to taste
- Optional toppings (avocado, vegan sour cream, green onions)

Preparation:

1. In a large pot, sauté onion and garlic until softened.
2. Add diced tomatoes, kidney beans, black beans, corn, chili powder, cumin, paprika, oregano, and salt and pepper to the pot. Stir to combine.
3. Let the chili simmer for 30 minutes, stirring occasionally.
4. Serve hot with toppings of choice.

Sweet Potato and Black Bean Enchiladas:

Cook time: 45 minutes

Serving: 4

Ingredients:

- 8 tortillas
- 2 sweet potatoes, diced

- 1 can black beans, drained and rinsed
- 1 bell pepper, diced
- 1 onion, diced
- 1 tsp cumin
- 1 tsp chili powder
- 1 tsp garlic powder
- Salt and pepper to taste
- 1 jar enchilada sauce
- 1 cup shredded vegan cheese
- Optional toppings (avocado, cilantro, salsa)

Preparation:
1. Preheat oven to 375°F (190°C).
2. In a pan over medium heat, sauté sweet potatoes, black beans, bell pepper, and onion until softened.
3. Add cumin, chili powder, garlic powder, salt, and pepper to the pan and stir to combine.
4. Warm tortillas in another pan over low heat.
5. In a baking dish, spread a thin layer of enchilada sauce on the bottom.
6. Fill each tortilla with the sweet potato and black bean mixture and roll up. Place the enchiladas in the baking dish, seam-side down.
7. Pour the remaining enchilada sauce over the enchiladas.
8. Sprinkle shredded vegan cheese over the top and cover with foil.
9. Bake for 20 minutes, then remove the foil and bake for an additional 10 minutes.
10. Serve hot with desired toppings.

Quinoa-Stuffed Acorn Squash

Cook time: 1 hour

Serving: 4

Ingredients:
- 2 acorn squash, halved and seeded
- 1 cup quinoa
- 1 can black beans, drained and rinsed
- 1 bell pepper, diced
- 1 onion, diced
- 1 tsp cumin

- 1 tsp chili powder
- 1 tsp garlic powder
- Salt and pepper to taste
- Optional toppings (avocado, vegan sour cream, cilantro)

Preparation:
1. Preheat oven to 400°F (200°C).
2. Place acorn squash halves on a baking sheet and roast for 30 minutes, or until tender.
3. In a pot, cook quinoa according to package instructions.
4. In a pan over medium heat, sauté bell pepper and onion until softened.
5. Add black beans, cumin, chili powder, garlic powder, salt, and pepper to the pan with the vegetables. Cook for 5 minutes.
6. Stir the cooked quinoa into the black bean and vegetable mixture.
7. Fill each acorn squash half with the quinoa and black bean mixture.
8. Bake for an additional 15 minutes.
9. Serve hot with desired toppings.

Mushroom Risotto

Cook time: 40 minutes
Serving: 4
Ingredients:
- 1 cup Arborio rice
- 4 cups vegetable broth
- 1 onion, diced
- 2 cloves garlic, minced
- 8 oz mushrooms, sliced
- 1 tsp thyme
- 1 tsp rosemary
- 1 tsp sage
- Salt and pepper to taste
- 1/4 cup vegan butter
- Vegan Parmesan cheese

Preparation:
1. In a pot, heat vegetable broth over medium-low heat.

2. In another pot, melt vegan butter over medium heat. Add onion and garlic and sauté until softened.
3. Add Arborio rice to the pot with the onions and garlic, stirring constantly for about 2 minutes.
4. Reduce heat to medium and add a ladleful of vegetable broth to the pot, stirring until the liquid is absorbed.
5. Continue adding vegetable broth, one ladleful at a time, and stirring until the rice is cooked and creamy (about 20-25 minutes).
6. In a separate pan, sauté mushrooms until tender.
7. Stir mushrooms, thyme, rosemary, sage, salt, and pepper into the risotto.
8. Serve hot, topped with vegan Parmesan cheese.

Chapter 7: Tasty Snacks

Mixed Nuts

Cook time: 15 minutes

Serving: 2 cups

Ingredients:

- 1 cup almonds
- 1 cup cashews
- 1 cup walnuts
- 1 cup pecans
- 1 tablespoon butter
- 1 teaspoon salt
- 1 teaspoon garlic powder
- 1 teaspoon dried rosemary
- 1/4 teaspoon cayenne pepper

Preparation:

1. Preheat your oven to 350°F (180°C).
2. In a bowl, mix all the nuts together.
3. Melt butter in a microwave-safe bowl, then mix in the salt, garlic powder, dried rosemary, and cayenne pepper.
4. Pour the butter mixture over the nuts and toss to coat evenly.

5. Spread the nuts on a baking sheet and bake in the oven for 10-12 minutes, stirring once halfway through.
6. Let the nuts cool before serving. Store any leftovers in an airtight container for up to a week.

Air-Popped Popcorn

Cook time: 5 minutes

Serving: 2 servings

Ingredients:

- 1/4 cup of popcorn kernels
- 1 tablespoon of olive oil
- Salt to taste

Preparation:

1. In a small bowl, mix together the popcorn kernels and olive oil.
2. Place the mixture in a brown paper bag and fold the top twice to seal it.
3. Microwave for 2 minutes and 30 seconds, or until the popping slows down to 2 seconds per pop.
4. Add salt to taste and shake the bag to coat the popcorn evenly.
5. Enjoy as a low-calorie and fiber-rich snack.

Veggie Sticks with Hummus

Cook time: 10 minutes

Serving: 2 people

Ingredients:

- 1 red bell pepper
- 1 yellow bell pepper
- 2 carrots
- 2 celery stalks
- 1 cucumber
- 1 cup hummus

Preparation:

1. Wash and dry all vegetables.
2. Cut the bell peppers, carrots, celery, and cucumber into long, thin sticks.
3. Arrange the veggie sticks on a plate or in a container for easy serving.

4. Scoop the hummus into a small bowl and place it in the center of the veggie sticks platter.

5. Serve and enjoy as a healthy snack or appetizer. Optional: add additional veggies of your choice such as cherry tomatoes or broccoli florets.

Greek Yogurt with Berries

Cook time: 5 minutes

Serving: 1

Ingredients:

- 1/2 cup plain Greek yogurt
- 1/4 cup mixed berries (strawberries, blueberries, raspberries)
- 1 tablespoon honey
- 1 tablespoon chopped nuts (optional)
- 1 teaspoon chia seeds (optional)

Preparation:

1. In a small bowl, mix together the Greek yogurt and honey.
2. Wash and chop the berries and add them to the yogurt mixture.
3. Top with chopped nuts and chia seeds, if desired.
4. Mix everything together well and enjoy immediately. Serve cold.

Edamame

Cook time: 5 minutes

Serving: 1 serving

Ingredients:

- 1/2 cup of frozen edamame
- Salt to taste
- Optional seasonings (garlic powder, chili powder, etc.)

Preparation:

1. Cook the frozen edamame according to package instructions.
2. Drain and rinse the edamame.
3. Add salt and optional seasonings to taste, and mix well.
4. Enjoy as a protein-rich and flavorful snack.

Cottage Cheese with Pineapple

Cook time: 5 minutes

Serving: 2

Ingredients:

- 1 cup cottage cheese
- 1/2 cup diced pineapple
- 1 tablespoon honey
- 1/4 teaspoon cinnamon

Preparation:

1. In a small mixing bowl, combine cottage cheese, diced pineapple, honey, and cinnamon.
2. Stir until well combined.
3. Serve immediately or refrigerate until ready to serve.
4. Optional: Sprinkle with additional cinnamon on top for extra flavor. Enjoy your Cottage Cheese with Pineapple!

Sliced Apple with Almond Butter

Cook time: 5 minutes

Serving: 1-2

Ingredients:

- 1 apple
- 2 tablespoons almond butter
- Optional toppings: cinnamon, honey, chopped nuts

Preparation:

1. Wash and core the apple, then slice it into thin rounds.
2. Spread almond butter on each apple slice.
3. Optional: sprinkle cinnamon on top for extra flavor.
4. Optional: drizzle honey on top for added sweetness.
5. Optional: sprinkle chopped nuts on top for added crunch.
6. Serve and enjoy! This snack can be kept in the fridge for later consumption.

Rice Cakes with Avocado

Cook time: 10 minutes

Serving: 2

Ingredients:

- 2 rice cakes
- 1 avocado
- 1 tablespoon olive oil
- Salt and pepper to taste
- Optional toppings: sliced cherry tomatoes, sliced cucumbers, feta cheese, red pepper flakes

Preparation:

1. Begin by halving the avocado and removing the pit. Slice the avocado into thin pieces.
2. Heat olive oil in a skillet over medium heat.
3. Add the rice cakes to the skillet and cook for 2-3 minutes on each side, until lightly toasted.
4. Transfer the rice cakes to a serving plate and sprinkle with salt and pepper.
5. Top each rice cake with sliced avocado.
6. Add any additional toppings of your choice, such as sliced cherry tomatoes, cucumbers, feta cheese, or red pepper flakes.
7. Serve and enjoy your delicious rice cakes with avocado! You can also add a sprinkle of lemon juice for extra flavor.

Trail Mix

Cook time: None

Serving: 4 people

Ingredients:

- 1 cup of roasted peanuts
- 1 cup of almonds
- 1 cup of cashews
- 1 cup of dried cranberries
- 1 cup of dark chocolate chips

Preparation:

1. In a large bowl, mix together the roasted peanuts, almonds, cashews, and dried cranberries.
2. Add in the dark chocolate chips and mix well.
3. Store the trail mix in an airtight container or divided into individual serving bags.
4. Enjoy as a snack on-the-go, during hikes, or for a quick energy boost during the day. Enjoy!

Baked Sweet Potato Fries

Cook time: 25 minutes

Serving: 2 servings

Ingredients:

- 1 sweet potato, cut into matchsticks
- 1 tablespoon of olive oil
- Salt and pepper to taste

Preparation:

1. Preheat oven to 400 degrees Fahrenheit (200 degrees Celsius).
2. In a bowl, coat the sweet potato matchsticks with olive oil, salt, and pepper.
3. Spread the sweet potato fries on a baking sheet lined with parchment paper.
4. Bake for 20-25 minutes, flipping halfway through, until crispy.
5. Enjoy as a nutritious and guilt-free snack.

Chapter 8: Dessert Indulgences

Berry Sorbet

Cook time: 2 hours (including freezing time)

Serving: 4

Ingredients:

- 2 cups frozen mixed berries

- 1/4 cup honey
- 1/4 cup fresh lemon juice
- 1/2 cup water

Preparation:
1. In a blender, combine frozen berries, honey, lemon juice, and water. Blend until smooth.
2. Place the mixture in a loaf pan and freeze for about 2 hours, until solid.
3. When ready to serve, let the sorbet sit at room temperature for 5-10 minutes, then scoop and enjoy!

Dark Chocolate-Dipped Strawberries

Cook time: 15 minutes

Serving: 12

Ingredients:
- 12 fresh strawberries
- 1 cup dark chocolate chips
- 1 tablespoon coconut oil

Preparation:
1. Rinse and dry the strawberries.
2. In a double boiler, melt the dark chocolate chips and coconut oil until smooth.
3. Dip each strawberry into the chocolate, making sure it's completely covered.
4. Place the strawberries on a parchment-lined baking sheet and let them set in the fridge for about 10 minutes.
5. Serve and enjoy!

Baked Apples with Cinnamon

Cook time: 30 minutes

Serving: 4

Ingredients:
- 4 apples
- 1/4 cup honey
- 1 teaspoon cinnamon

- 1/4 cup chopped nuts of your choice

Preparation:
1. Preheat the oven to 375°F (190°C).
2. Core the apples and place them in a baking dish.
3. In a small bowl, mix together honey and cinnamon.
4. Drizzle the honey-cinnamon mixture over the apples, making sure to cover them evenly.
5. Sprinkle the chopped nuts on top of the apples.
6. Bake for 30 minutes, or until the apples are soft.
7. Serve warm and enjoy as is or with a scoop of vanilla ice cream.

Greek Yogurt Parfait with Honey and Granola

Cook time: 10 minutes

Serving: 2

Ingredients:
- 1 cup plain Greek yogurt
- 2 tablespoons honey
- 1/2 cup granola
- 1/2 cup mixed berries

Preparation:
1. In a small bowl, mix together Greek yogurt and honey.
2. In a glass or bowl, layer the yogurt, granola, and berries.
3. Repeat layering until all ingredients are used up.
4. Serve and enjoy!

Chia Seed Pudding with Mango

Cook time: 4 hours (or overnight)

Serving: 2

Ingredients:
- 1/4 cup chia seeds
- 1 cup unsweetened almond milk
- 1 tablespoon honey
- 1/2 teaspoon vanilla extract
- 1 mango, diced

Preparation:

1. In a small bowl, whisk together chia seeds, almond milk, honey, and vanilla extract.
2. Cover and refrigerate for at least 4 hours or overnight.
3. Once the chia pudding has set, top with diced mango and serve.

Chocolate Avocado Mousse

Cook time: 10 minutes

Serving: 2

Ingredients:

- 2 ripe avocados
- 1/4 cup cocoa powder
- 1/4 cup honey
- 1/4 cup unsweetened almond milk

Preparation:

1. Scoop out the flesh of the avocados and place them in a blender or food processor.
2. Add in cocoa powder, honey, and almond milk. Blend until smooth and creamy.
3. Serve immediately or refrigerate until ready to serve.

Frozen Banana Bites

Cook time: 1 hour (including freezing time)

Serving: 4

Ingredients:

- 2 ripe bananas
- 1/4 cup peanut butter
- 1/4 cup dark chocolate chips
- 1 tablespoon coconut oil

Preparation:

1. Slice the bananas into thin rounds.
2. Place a dollop of peanut butter on half of the banana rounds and top with the remaining rounds.

3. Place them on a baking sheet lined with parchment paper and freeze for about 30 minutes.
4. In a double boiler, melt the dark chocolate chips and coconut oil until smooth.
5. Dip each frozen banana bite into the melted chocolate and place them back on the baking sheet.
6. Freeze for another 30 minutes, until the chocolate has hardened.
7. Serve and enjoy!

Almond Flour Brownies

Cook time: 30 minutes

Serving: 9

Ingredients:
- 1 cup almond flour
- 1/3 cup cocoa powder
- 1/4 teaspoon baking soda
- 1/4 teaspoon salt
- 1/4 cup honey
- 3 tablespoons coconut oil, melted
- 2 eggs
- 1 teaspoon vanilla extract

Preparation:
1. Preheat the oven to 350°F (175°C).
2. In a mixing bowl, combine almond flour, cocoa powder, baking soda, and salt.
3. In a separate bowl, whisk together honey, coconut oil, eggs, and vanilla extract.
4. Pour the wet ingredients into the dry ingredients and mix until well combined.
5. Pour the batter into a greased 8x8 inch baking dish and bake for 25-30 minutes, until a toothpick inserted in the middle comes out clean.
6. Let the brownies cool before slicing and serving.

Rice Pudding with Raisins

Cook time: 30 minutes

Serving: 4

Ingredients:

- 1 cup cooked white rice
- 2 cups milk
- 1/4 cup honey
- 1/4 teaspoon cinnamon
- 1/4 cup raisins

Preparation:

1. In a saucepan, combine cooked rice, milk, honey, and cinnamon. Bring to a simmer over medium heat.
2. Cook for about 20 minutes, stirring occasionally, until the mixture has thickened.
3. Stir in raisins and cook for another 5 minutes.
4. Serve warm or chilled, depending on preference.

Lemon Poppy Seed Muffins

Cook time: 25 minutes

Serving: 12

Ingredients:

- 2 cups almond flour
- 1/3 cup honey
- 1/4 cup coconut oil, melted
- 2 eggs
- 1/4 cup fresh lemon juice
- 2 tablespoons poppy seeds
- 1 teaspoon lemon zest
- 1 teaspoon baking soda
- 1/2 teaspoon salt

Preparation:

1. Preheat the oven to 350°F (175°C).
2. In a mixing bowl, whisk together almond flour, honey, coconut oil, eggs, lemon juice, poppy seeds, lemon zest, baking soda, and salt.
3. Pour the batter into a greased muffin tin, filling each cup about 3/4 full.
4. Bake for 20-25 minutes, until a toothpick inserted in the middle comes out clean.

5. Let the muffins cool before serving.

Chapter 9: Hydrating Beverages

Infused Water with Citrus and Mint

Cook time: 5 minutes

Serving: 1 pitcher

Ingredients:

- 1 large pitcher of water
- 1 lemon, sliced
- 1 lime, sliced
- 1 orange, sliced
- 10-12 fresh mint leaves

Preparation:

1. In the pitcher, add water and sliced citrus fruits.
2. Gently crush the mint leaves with your hands and add them to the pitcher.
3. Stir gently to release the flavor of the fruits and mint.
4. Let the water sit for at least 30 minutes for the flavors to infuse.
5. Serve over ice and garnish with extra citrus slices and mint leaves, if desired.

Green Tea

Cook time: 5 minutes

Serving: 1 cup

Ingredients:

- 1 green tea bag
- 1 cup of boiling water
- 1 tsp honey (optional)

Preparation:

1. Place the green tea bag in a mug.

2. Pour the boiling water over the tea bag and let it steep for 3-5 minutes.
3. Remove the tea bag and stir in honey, if desired.
4. Let the tea cool down before serving, or serve over ice for iced green tea.

Herbal Tea

Cook time: 5 minutes

Serving: 1 cup

Ingredients:

- 1 herbal tea bag (such as chamomile, peppermint, or ginger)
- 1 cup of boiling water
- 1 tsp honey (optional)

Preparation:

1. Place the herbal tea bag in a mug.
2. Pour the boiling water over the tea bag and let it steep according to the recommended time on the packaging.
3. Remove the tea bag and stir in honey, if desired.
4. Let the tea cool down before serving, or serve over ice for iced herbal tea.

Fresh Fruit Smoothie

Cook time: 5 minutes

Serving: 1 large glass

Ingredients:

- 1 banana, sliced
- 1 cup of frozen berries
- 1 cup of almond milk
- 1 tbsp honey

Preparation:

1. Place all ingredients in a blender.
2. Blend until smooth.
3. If the smoothie is too thick, add more almond milk. If it's too thin, add more frozen berries.
4. Pour into a glass and serve immediately.

Iced Coffee with Almond Milk

Cook time: 5 minutes

Serving: 1 glass

Ingredients:

- 1 cup of cold brew coffee (or 1 cup of brewed coffee, cooled in the fridge)
- 1/4 cup of almond milk
- 1 tsp honey (optional)

Preparation:

1. In a glass, mix together the coffee and almond milk.
2. Add honey, if desired.
3. Serve over ice for a refreshing iced coffee.

Coconut Water

Cook time: 5 minutes

Serving: 1

Ingredients:

- 1 cup coconut water
- 1/2 lime, juiced
- 1 tsp honey
- 1/4 tsp sea salt
- Ice cubes

Preparation:

1. In a glass, combine coconut water, lime juice, honey, and sea salt.
2. Stir until well combined.
3. Add ice cubes and serve immediately.

Cucumber and Mint Cooler

Cook time: 10 minutes

Serving: 1

Ingredients:

- 1 cup sparkling water
- 1/4 cup cucumber, sliced
- 4 mint leaves
- 1 tsp agave syrup

- Ice cubes

Preparation:
1. In a glass, muddle the cucumber slices and mint leaves together.
2. Add sparkling water and agave syrup, and stir until well combined.
3. Add ice cubes and serve chilled.

Ginger Lemonade

Cook time: 15 minutes

Serving: 2

Ingredients:
- 1/2 cup freshly squeezed lemon juice
- 1/4 cup honey
- 1-inch piece of ginger, peeled and sliced
- 2 cups water
- Ice cubes

Preparation:
1. In a small pot, bring water to a simmer and add ginger slices.
2. Let simmer for 10 minutes and then remove from heat.
3. Add honey and stir until dissolved.
4. Let mixture cool, then strain out ginger slices.
5. In a pitcher, combine the ginger lemon mixture and lemon juice.
6. Chill in the refrigerator for at least 1 hour.
7. Serve over ice and enjoy!

Sparkling Water with Berries

Cook time: 5 minutes

Serving: 1

Ingredients:
- 1 cup sparkling water
- 1/4 cup mixed berries (such as strawberries, blueberries, and raspberries)
- 1 tbsp honey
- 1 tbsp lemon juice
- Ice cubes

Preparation:

1. In a glass, muddle the mixed berries until slightly crushed.
2. Add honey and lemon juice to the glass and stir until well combined.
3. Pour in sparkling water and stir.
4. Add ice cubes and serve chilled.

Watermelon Slushie

Cook time: 5 minutes

Serving: 2

Ingredients:

- 2 cups watermelon, cubed
- 1/2 cup coconut water
- Juice from 1 lime
- 1 tsp honey
- Ice cubes

Preparation:

- In a blender, combine watermelon, coconut water, lime juice, and honey.
- Blend until smooth.
- Pour mixture into glasses filled with ice cubes.
- Serve immediately and enjoy your refreshing Watermelon Slushie.

Chapter 10: Noom-Friendly Comfort Food

Cauliflower Mac and Cheese

Cook time: 40 minutes

Serving: 6

Ingredients:

- 1 head of cauliflower
- 2 cups of elbow macaroni
- 2 tablespoons of butter

- 2 tablespoons of all-purpose flour
- 1 cup of milk
- 1 cup of shredded cheddar cheese
- Salt and pepper to taste

Preparation:
1. Preheat your oven to 375 degrees Fahrenheit.
2. Cut the cauliflower into small florets and boil them in a pot of salted water for 5 minutes.
3. Cook the macaroni according to package instructions, drain, and set aside.
4. In a separate saucepan, melt the butter over medium heat. Add in the flour and whisk until smooth.
5. Slowly pour in the milk, whisking continuously until the mixture thickens.
6. Remove the saucepan from heat and stir in the shredded cheese until fully melted.
7. Season with salt and pepper to taste.
8. In a greased 9x13 inch baking dish, mix together the cooked macaroni, cauliflower, and cheese sauce.
9. Bake in the preheated oven for 20-25 minutes, or until the top is golden brown.
10. Serve and enjoy your delicious and healthier version of mac and cheese.

Turkey and Vegetable Pot Pie

Cook time: 45 minutes

Serving: 4

Ingredients:
- 1 tablespoon of olive oil
- 1 onion, chopped
- 2 cloves of garlic, minced
- 1 cup of diced carrots
- 1 cup of diced celery
- 1 cup of diced potatoes
- 1 pound of ground turkey
- 1/2 cup of chicken broth
- 1/2 cup of frozen peas
- 1 teaspoon of dried thyme
- Salt and pepper to taste

- 1 pie crust

Preparation:
1. Preheat your oven to 375 degrees Fahrenheit.
2. In a large skillet, heat the olive oil over medium heat. Add in the onion and garlic and cook for 2-3 minutes until softened.
3. Add in the carrots, celery, and potatoes and cook for another 5 minutes.
4. Add in the ground turkey and continue cooking until it is fully cooked.
5. Pour in the chicken broth and stir in the frozen peas and dried thyme. Let simmer for 5 minutes.
6. Season with salt and pepper to taste.
7. Transfer the mixture into a 9-inch pie dish.
8. Place the pie crust on top of the mixture, crimping the edges to seal it.
9. Cut a few slits in the top of the crust to allow steam to escape.
10. Bake for 25-30 minutes, or until the crust is golden brown. Serve and enjoy your hearty and healthy pot pie.

Spaghetti Squash with Marinara

Cook time: 45 minutes

Serving: 4

Ingredients:
- 1 large spaghetti squash
- 1 tablespoon of olive oil
- 1 onion, chopped
- 2 cloves of garlic, minced
- 1 can of diced tomatoes
- 1 teaspoon of dried oregano
- 1 teaspoon of dried basil
- Salt and pepper to taste
- Grated parmesan cheese for serving (optional)

Preparation:
1. Preheat your oven to 400 degrees Fahrenheit.
2. Cut the spaghetti squash in half lengthwise and scoop out the seeds. Rub olive oil on the flesh of the squash and place face-down on a baking sheet.
3. Bake the squash for 30-40 minutes, or until the flesh is easily pierced with a fork.

4. While the squash is baking, heat the olive oil in a saucepan over medium heat. Add in the onion and garlic and cook for 2-3 minutes until softened.
5. Stir in the canned tomatoes, dried oregano, and dried basil. Let simmer for 10-15 minutes.
6. Season with salt and pepper to taste.
7. Once the spaghetti squash is cooked, use a fork to scrape out the flesh, creating the "spaghetti" strands.
8. Serve the squash with the marinara sauce on top. Optional: sprinkle with grated parmesan cheese for extra flavor. Enjoy your low-carb and nutritious spaghetti alternative.

Baked Chicken Tenders

Cook time: 25 minutes

Serving: 4

Ingredients:

- 1 pound of chicken tenders
- 1/2 cup of flour
- 1/2 teaspoon of garlic powder
- 1/2 teaspoon of onion powder
- Salt and pepper to taste
- 2 eggs, beaten
- 1 cup of breadcrumbs
- Cooking spray

Preparation:

1. Preheat your oven to 375 degrees Fahrenheit.
2. In a shallow dish, mix together the flour, garlic powder, onion powder, salt, and pepper.
3. In another shallow dish, beat the eggs.
4. In a third shallow dish, add the breadcrumbs.
5. Dredge the chicken tenders in the flour mixture, then dip them in the beaten eggs, and finally coat them in the breadcrumbs.
6. Place the coated tenders on a greased baking sheet.
7. Spray the tenders with cooking spray to give them a crispy texture.
8. Bake in the preheated oven for 20-25 minutes, or until the chicken is cooked through and the coating is crispy.

9. Serve with your choice of dipping sauce and enjoy your healthier version of chicken tenders.

Quinoa-Stuffed Bell Peppers

Cook time: 45 minutes

Serving: 4

Ingredients:

- 4 bell peppers
- 1 cup of quinoa
- 2 cups of vegetable broth
- 1 can of black beans, drained and rinsed
- 1 can of corn, drained
- 1 cup of shredded cheddar cheese
- 1 teaspoon of cumin
- 1 teaspoon of chili powder
- Salt and pepper to taste

Preparation:

1. Preheat your oven to 375 degrees Fahrenheit.
2. Cut the tops off of the bell peppers and remove the seeds inside.
3. In a saucepan, bring the quinoa and vegetable broth to a boil. Reduce the heat and let it simmer for 15-20 minutes, or until all the liquid is absorbed.
4. In a large bowl, mix together the cooked quinoa, black beans, corn, shredded cheese, cumin, chili powder, salt, and pepper.
5. Stuff the mixture into the hollowed-out bell peppers.
6. Place the stuffed peppers in a baking dish and bake for 20-25 minutes, or until the peppers are soft and the filling is heated through.
7. Serve and enjoy your nutritious and delicious quinoa-stuffed bell peppers.

Black Bean and Corn Quesadilla

Cook time: 15 minutes

Serving: 4

Ingredients:

- 8 small flour tortillas
- 1 can of black beans, drained and rinsed
- 1 can of corn, drained

- 1/2 cup of diced bell pepper
- 1/2 cup of diced onion
- 1 cup of shredded cheddar cheese
- 1 teaspoon of cumin
- 1 teaspoon of chili powder
- Salt and pepper to taste

Preparation:
1. In a bowl, mix together the black beans, corn, diced bell pepper, diced onion, shredded cheese, cumin, chili powder, salt, and pepper.
2. Heat a large non-stick skillet over medium heat. Place one tortilla in the skillet.
3. On one half of the tortilla, spread an even layer of the bean and corn mixture. Fold the other half of the tortilla over the filling.
4. Cook for 2-3 minutes on each side, or until the tortilla is crispy and the cheese is melted.
5. Repeat with the remaining tortillas and filling.
6. Serve and enjoy your tasty and protein-packed black bean and corn quesadillas.

Turkey and Mushroom Stroganoff

Cook time: 30 minutes

Serving: 4

Ingredients:
- 1 pound of ground turkey
- 1 tablespoon of olive oil
- 1 onion, chopped
- 2 cloves of garlic, minced
- 8 ounces of sliced mushrooms
- 1 cup of beef broth
- 1/2 cup of sour cream
- 1 tablespoon of dijon mustard
- 1 tablespoon of Worcestershire sauce
- Salt and pepper to taste
- 8 ounces of egg noodles

Preparation:

1. In a large skillet, cook the ground turkey over medium heat until fully cooked. Set aside.
2. In the same skillet, heat the olive oil over medium heat. Add in the onion and garlic and cook for 2-3 minutes until softened.
3. Add in the sliced mushrooms and cook for another 5 minutes.
4. Pour in the beef broth, sour cream, dijon mustard, and Worcestershire sauce. Stir until well combined.
5. Add the cooked ground turkey back into the skillet and let simmer for 10-15 minutes.
6. Season with salt and pepper to taste.
7. While the stroganoff is simmering, cook the egg noodles according to package instructions.
8. Serve the stroganoff on top of the egg noodles and enjoy your hearty and flavorful meal.

Sweet Potato and Black Bean Burger

Cook time: 30 minutes

Serving: 4

Ingredients:

- 2 medium sweet potatoes, peeled and cubed
- 1 can of black beans, drained and rinsed
- 1/4 cup of breadcrumbs
- 1/4 cup of diced onion
- 2 cloves of garlic, minced
- 1 teaspoon of cumin
- 1 teaspoon of chili powder
- Salt and pepper to taste
- 4 whole grain burger buns
- Lettuce, tomato, and other desired toppings

Preparation:

1. Preheat your oven to 375 degrees Fahrenheit.
2. In a pot of boiling water, cook the cubed sweet potatoes for 10-15 minutes, or until soft.
3. In a large bowl, mash the cooked sweet potatoes and black beans together with a potato masher or fork.

4. Add in the breadcrumbs, diced onion, minced garlic, cumin, chili powder, salt, and pepper. Mix until well combined.
5. Form the mixture into four evenly sized patties.
6. Place the patties on a greased baking sheet and bake for 20-25 minutes, flipping halfway through.
7. Serve on whole grain burger buns with your desired toppings. Enjoy your tasty and nutritious sweet potato and black bean burgers.

Baked Zucchini Fries

Cook time: 20 minutes

Serving: 4

Ingredients:

- 2 zucchinis, cut into thin strips
- 1/2 cup of flour
- 2 eggs, beaten
- 1 cup of breadcrumbs
- 1/4 cup of grated parmesan cheese
- 1/2 teaspoon of garlic powder
- Salt and pepper to taste
- Cooking spray
- Marinara sauce for dipping (optional)

Preparation:

1. Preheat your oven to 400 degrees Fahrenheit.
2. Line a baking sheet with parchment paper.
3. Place the flour in a shallow dish, the beaten eggs in another shallow dish, and the breadcrumbs, grated parmesan cheese, garlic powder, salt, and pepper in a third shallow dish.
4. Toss the zucchini strips in the flour, then dip them in the beaten eggs, and finally coat them in the breadcrumb mixture.
5. Place the coated zucchini strips on the prepared baking sheet.
6. Spray the zucchini fries with cooking spray to give them a crispy texture.
7. Bake for 15-20 minutes, or until the zucchini is tender and the coating is golden brown.
8. Serve with marinara sauce for dipping, if desired. Enjoy your healthier version of French fries.

Veggie and Lentil Shepherd's Pie

Cook time: 50 minutes

Serving: 4

Ingredients:

- 1/2 cup of dried green lentils
- 1 tablespoon of olive oil
- 1 onion, chopped
- 2 cloves of garlic, minced
- 2 carrots, diced
- 2 stalks of celery, diced
- 1 cup of frozen peas
- 1 can of corn, drained
- 2 tablespoons of all-purpose flour
- 1 cup of vegetable broth
- 1 tablespoon of tomato paste
- 1 teaspoon of dried thyme
- Salt and pepper to taste
- 4 cups of mashed potatoes

Preparation:

1. Preheat your oven to 375 degrees Fahrenheit.
2. Cook the lentils according to package instructions and set aside.
3. In a large skillet, heat the olive oil over medium heat. Add in the onion and garlic and cook for 2-3 minutes until softened.
4. Add in the diced carrots and celery and cook for another 5 minutes.
5. Stir in the cooked lentils, frozen peas, and canned corn.
6. Sprinkle the flour over the mixture and stir to combine.
7. Slowly pour in the vegetable broth and stir in the tomato paste and dried thyme. Let simmer for 10-15 minutes.
8. Season with salt and pepper to taste.
9. In a 9x13 inch baking dish, spread an even layer of the lentil and vegetable mixture. Top with the mashed potatoes.
10. Bake for 20-25 minutes, or until the mashed potatoes are lightly golden. Serve and enjoy your hearty and filling shepherd's pie.